The ABC's of Mental Health, Suicide & Domestic Violence

The ABC's of Mental Health, Suicide & Domestic Violence

Temeka Jefferson

Superior Publishing LLC.

I would like to honor and dedicate this book to
Desmond Chandler (1/30/78-1/8/92)

From the Author

Pay attention to your loved ones behavior and persona. If you notice they aren't their normal self seek help and continue to follow up. This may just save their life. Not all acts are just attention seeking but indeed a cry for help.

A

Always ask for help

B

Believe in yourself!

BREAK FREE

C

Continue to fight/
courageous

D

Don't give up!

Don't count yourself out!

E

Every day is a new day.

F

Fight with all your might!

G

Give it your all!

H

Happy Thoughts

I

Include & involve others

I'm a BIG deal

J

Just hang in there.

K

Keep striving

L

Love yourself

M

Make baby steps

N

Never forget you
are needed &
loved

O

Ongoing strength

P

Patience is the key!

PUSH THROUGH

Q

*Quitting is
not an option!*

R

Remind yourself
you are great.

S

STAY STRONG

T

The world needs you.

U

Uniquely you
Use your voice

V

Value yourself!
Venting is good.

W

Wonderfully made

XOXO

HUGS & KISSES

Y

You are not alone.

Z

Zero tolerance

H.O.P.E.

HOPE

HELPING OTHER PEOPLE ENDURE

Temeka Jefferson, is the granddaughter of the late Nathaniel and Leona Jefferson and the late Fred and Nettie Davidson. She is the daughter of Sammie and Nettie Jefferson Sr. She is the fourth of five children. Jefferson is a 1998 graduate of West Point High School and graduate of Mississippi State University and Bel-haven University in receiving her a double Master.

She is a Certified Mental Therapist and being a Therapist is her greatest passion of over 20 years. At age 12 she lost a dear loved one to suicide in which she was prompt to become a therapist. She dedicates this book in honor of him, Desmond Chandler.

Temeka grew up on a farm, caring for her father's animals, especially his Tennessee Walking horses, therefore; she and her family traveled the world. Dealing with horses and being a therapist both play a major role in her life today. Since being a Therapist, she has worked with several populations: domestic violence, suicidal and several that have been diagnosed with mental health issues/disorders.

Thank You
I would like to thank GOD, my family and friends for walking this journey with me.
With God all things are possible.

www.ingramcontent.com/pod-product-compliance
Lightning Source LLC
Chambersburg PA
CBRC101142030426
42335CB00007B/204